The Complete Keto Slow Cooker Cookbook

Over 50 Best Recipes You Must Try

Elena Johnson

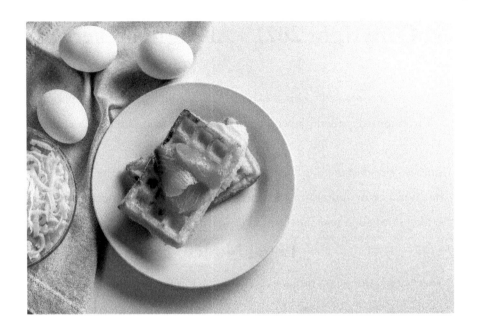

TABLE OF CONTENTS

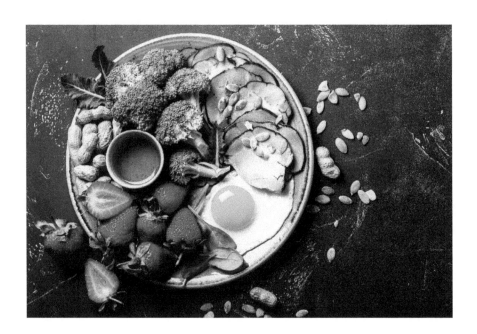

INTRODUCTION

The ketogenic diet is trendy, and for an excellent reason. It truly teaches healthy eating without forcing anyone into at risk. The success rate of keto is relatively high. While there are no specific numbers to suggest the exact rate, it is only fair to state that those who have the will to change their lifestyle and are okay adjusting to new eating habits, almost every one of them will make it through as a success story.

A diet that results in the production of ketone bodies by the liver is called a ketogenic diet; it causes your system to use fat instead of carbohydrates for energy. Limit your carbohydrate intake to a low level, causing some reactions. However, it is not a high protein diet. It involves moderate protein, low carbohydrate intake, and high fat intake.

Regardless of your lifestyle, everyone benefits from the keto diet in the following ways:

Weight Loss

Far more important than the visual aspect of excess weight is its negative influence on your body. Too much weight affects the efficiency of your body's blood flow, which in turn also affects how much oxygen your heart is able to pump to every part of your system. Too much weight also means that there are layers of fat covering your internal organs, which prevents them from working efficiently. It makes it hard to walk because it puts great pressure on your joints, and makes it very difficult to complete even regular daily tasks. A healthy weight allows your body to move freely and your entire internal system to work at its optimal levels.

Cognitive Focus

In order for your brain to function at its best, it needs to have balanced levels of all nutrients and molecules, because a balance allows it to focus on other things, such as working, studying, or creativity. If you eat carbs, the sudden insulin spike that comes with them will force your brain to stop whatever it was doing and to turn its focus on the correct breakdown of glucose molecules. This is why people often feel sleepy and with a foggy mind after high-carb meals. The keto diet keeps the balance strong, so that your brain does not have to deal with any sudden surprises.

Blood Sugar Control

If you already have diabetes, or are prone to it, then controlling your blood sugar is obviously of the utmost importance. However, even if you are not battling a type of diabetes at the moment, that doesn't mean that you are not in danger of developing it in the future. Most people forget that insulin is a finite resource in your body. You are given a certain amount of it, and it is gradually used up throughout your life. The more often you eat carbs, the more often your body needs to use insulin to break down the glucose; and when it reaches critically low levels of this finite resource, diabetes is formed.

Lower Cholesterol and Blood Pressure

Cholesterol and triglyceride levels maintain, or ruin, your arterial health. If your arteries are clogged up with cholesterol, they cannot efficiently transfer blood through your system, which in some cases even results in heart attacks. The keto diet keeps all of these levels at an optimal level, so that they do not interfere with your body's normal functioning.

Slow Cookers

Slow cookers are not new appliances in the culinary world. They have been around for decades; you might even have fond memories from your childhood of your parents serving your favorite dinner out of one. Slow cookers are very versatile because the cooking environment works the same no matter the cuisine. Knowing what slow cookers can and can't do is important for planning your meals, especially for a diet like keto.

Some of the reasons to use a slow cooker include:

Enhances flavor: Cooking ingredients over several hours with spices, herbs, and other seasonings creates vegetables and proteins that burst with delicious flavors. This slow process allows the flavors to mellow and deepen for an enhanced eating experience.

Saves time: Cooking at home takes a great deal of time: prepping, sautéing, stirring, turning the heat up and down, and watching the meal so that it does not over- or undercook. If you're unable to invest the time, you might find yourself reaching for convenience foods instead of healthy choices. Slow cookers allow you to do other activities while the meal cooks. You can put your ingredients in the slow cooker in the morning and come home to a perfectly cooked meal.

Convenient: Besides the time-saving aspect, using a slow cooker can free up the stove and oven for other dishes. This can be very convenient for large holiday meals or when you want to serve a side dish and entrée as well as a delectable dessert. Clean up is simple when you use the slow cooker for messy meals because most inserts are nonstick or are easily cleaned with a little soapy water, and each meal is prepared in either just the machine or using one additional vessel to sauté ingredients. There is no wide assortment of pots, pans, and baking dishes to contend with at the end of the day.

Low heat production: If you have ever cooked dinner on a scorching summer afternoon, you will appreciate the low amount of heat produced by a slow cooker. Even after eight hours of operation, slow cookers do not heat up your kitchen and you will not be sweating over the hot stovetop. Slow cookers use about a third of the energy of conventional cooking methods, just a little more energy than a traditional light bulb.

Supports healthy eating: Cooking your food at high heat can reduce the nutrition profile of your foods, breaking down and removing the majority of vitamins, minerals, and antioxidants while producing unhealthy chemical compounds that can contribute to disease. Low-heat cooking retains all the goodness that you want for your diet.

Saves Money: Slow cookers save you money because of the low amount of electricity they use and because the best ingredients for slow cooking are the less expensive cuts of beef and heartier inexpensive vegetables. Tougher cuts of meat—brisket, chuck, shanks—break down beautifully to fork-tender goodness. Another cost-saving benefit is that most 6-quart slow cookers will produce enough of a recipe to stretch your meals over at least two days. Leftovers are one of the best methods for saving money.

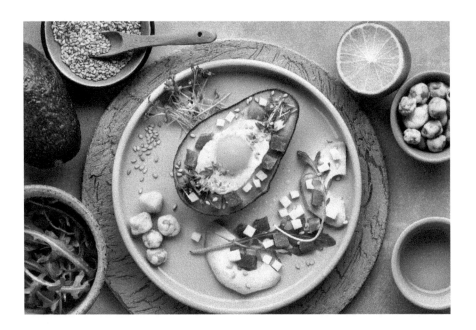

BREAKFAST

1. Breakfast Sweet Pepper Rounds

Preparation Time: 10 minutes

Cooking time: 3 hours

Servings: 4

Ingredients

- 2red sweet pepper
- 7oz.. ground chicken
- 5oz.. Parmesan
- 1tablespoon sour cream
- 1tablespoon flour
- 1egg
- 2teaspoon almond milk
- 1teaspoon salt
- 1/2teaspoon ground black pepper
- 1/4teaspoon butter

Directions:

1. Combine the sour cream with the ground chicken, flour, ground black pepper, almond milk, and butter.
2. Beat eggs into the mixture.
3. Detach the seeds from the sweet peppers and slice them roughly.

4. Place the pepper slices in the slow cooker and fill them with the ground chicken mixture.

5. After this, chop Parmesan into the cubes and add them to the sliced peppers.

6. Close and cook the dish for 3 hours on HIGH.

7. When the time is done make sure that the ground chicken is cooked and the cheese is melted. Enjoy the dish immediately.

Nutrition: Calories 261 Fat 8 Carbs 1.3 Protein 21

2. Breakfast Cauliflower Hash

Preparation Time: 17 minutes

Cooking time: 8 hours

Servings: 5

Ingredients:

- 7eggs
- 1/4cup milk
- 1teaspoon salt
- 1teaspoon ground black pepper
- 1/2teaspoon ground mustard
- 10oz.. cauliflower
- 1/4teaspoon chili flakes
- 5oz.. breakfast sausages, chopped
- 1/2onion, chopped
- 5oz.. Cheddar cheese, shredded

Directions:

1. Wash the cauliflower carefully and separate it into the florets.
2. After this, shred the cauliflower florets.
3. Beat the eggs and whisk. Add the milk, salt, ground black pepper, ground mustard, chili flakes, and chopped onion into the whisked egg mixture.
4. Put the shredded cauliflower in the slow cooker.
5. Add the whisked egg mixture. Add the shredded cheese and chopped sausages.

6. Stir the mixture gently and close the slow cooker lid.

7. Cook the dish on LOW for 8 hours. When the cauliflower hash is cooked, remove it from the slow cooker and mix up. Enjoy!

Nutrition: Calories 329 Fat 16 Carbs 1.0 Protein 23

3. <u>Savory Creamy Breakfast Casserole</u>

Preparation Time: 17 minutes

Cooking time: 5 hours on low / 3 hours on high

Servings: 5

Ingredients:

- 1tablespoon, extra-virgin olive oil
- 10large eggs, beaten
- 1cup heavy (whipping) cream
- 11/2cups shredded sharp Cheddar cheese, divided
- 1/2cup grated Romano cheese
- 1/2teaspoon kosher salt
- 1/4teaspoon freshly ground black pepper
- 8ounces thick-cut ham, diced
- 3/4 head broccoli, cut into small florets
- 1/2onion, diced

Directions:

1. Brush butter into a cooker.
2. Directly in the insert, whisk together the eggs, heavy cream, 1/2 cup of Cheddar cheese, the Romano cheese, salt, and pepper.
3. Stir in the ham, broccoli, and onion.
4. Cover and cook on low or 3 hours on high. Serve hot.

Nutrition: Calories 465 Fat 10 Carbs 5 Protein 28

4. Bacon & Cheese Frittata

Preparation Time: 15 minutes

Cooking time: 2 hours 30 minutes

Servings: 8

Ingredients:

- 1/2 lb.. bacon
- 2tablespoons butter
- 8oz.. fresh spinach, packed down
- 10eggs
- 1/2cup heavy whipping cream
- 1/2cup shredded cheese
- Salt and pepper

Directions:

1. Butter or grease the inside of your slow-cooker.
2. Loosely chop the spinach.
3. Cut bacon into half-inch pieces.
4. Beat the eggs with the spices, cream, cheese, and chopped spinach. Then everything will be blended smoothly.
5. Pour the egg mixture over the bacon.
6. Cover the slow cooker and adjust the temperature to high
7. Cook for 2 hours. Serve hot.

Nutrition: Calories 392 Fat 34 Carbs 4 Protein 19

5. Delight Breakfast Meatloaf

Preparation Time: 10 minutes

Cooking time: 3 hours 10 minutes

Servings: 8

Ingredients:

- 2lb.. ground pork
- 2 eggs
- 2tbsp.. paprika
- 2tbsp.. fresh sage
- 1tbsp.. olive oil
- 1diced onion
- 3garlic cloves
- 1/4cup of almond flour

Directions:

1. Saute vegetables in the slow cooker in the olive oil until brown.
2. Mix the pork, eggs, sage, paprika, and almond flour, thoroughly.
3. Add the cooked onions and garlic.
4. Put the loaf in the slow cooker, cover with the lid and cook for three hours on low heat.
5. Serve in slices immediately or save to serve at breakfast later.

Nutrition: Calories 406 Fat 26 Carbs 5 Protein 32

6. <u>Asparagus Smoked Salmon</u>

Preparation Time: 15 minutes

Cooking time: 5 hours

Servings: 6

Ingredients:

- 1tablespoon extra-virgin olive oil

- 6large eggs

- 1cup heavy (whipping) cream

- 2teaspoons chopped fresh dill, plus additional for garnish

- 1/2teaspoon kosher salt

- 1/4teaspoon freshly ground black pepper

- 11/2cups shredded Havarti or Monterey Jack cheese

- 12ounces asparagus, trimmed and sliced

- 6ounces smoked salmon, flaked

Directions:

1. Brush butter into a cooker

2. whisk in the heavy cream with eggs, dill, salt, and pepper.

3. Stir in the cheese and asparagus.

4. Gently fold in the salmon and then pour the mixture into the prepared insert.

5. Cover and cook on low or 3 hours on high.

6. Serve warm, garnished with additional fresh dill.

Nutrition: Calories 388 Fat 19 Carbs 1.0 Protein 21

LUNCH

7. Lemon Orzo

Preparation time: 20 minutes

Cooking time: 2 hours 30 minutes

Servings: 5

Ingredients:

- 4oz.. shallot
- 7oz.. orzo
- 2cup chicken stock
- 1teaspoon paprika
- 1teaspoon ground black pepper
- 1teaspoon salt
- 1lemon
- 1/4cup cream
- 2yellow sweet pepper
- 1cup baby spinach

Directions:

1. Chop the shallot and place it in the slow cooker.
2. Add the chicken stock and paprika. Sprinkle the mixture with the ground black pepper and salt. Stir it gently and cook on HIGH for 30 minutes.

3. Meanwhile, grate the zest from the lemon and squeeze the juice. Add the lemon zest and juice in the slow cooker and stir it. After this, chop the baby spinach.

4. Add it into the slow cooker. Remove the seeds from the yellow sweet peppers and chop into tiny pieces. Add the chopped peppers to the slow cooker.

5. Add orzo and heavy cream. Stir the mass carefully and close the slow cooker lid. Cook the dish for 2 hours on LOW. Mix the dish gently. Enjoy!

Nutrition: Calories 152, Fat 4, Fiber 3, Carbs 2.79, Protein 7

8. <u>Veggie Bean Stew</u>

Preparation time: 20 minutes

Cooking time: 7 hours

Servings: 8

Ingredients:

- 1/2cup barley
- 1cup black beans
- 1/4cup red beans
- 2carrots
- 1cup onion, chopped
- 1cup tomato juice
- 2potatoes
- 1teaspoon salt
- 1teaspoon ground black pepper
- 4cups water
- 4oz.. tofu
- 1teaspoon garlic powder
- 1cup fresh cilantro

Directions:

- Place barley, black beans, and red beans in the slow cooker vessel.
- Add chopped onion, tomato juice, salt, ground black pepper, and garlic powder. After this, add water and close the slow cooker lid.

- Cook the dish for 4 hours on HIGH.

- Meanwhile, peel the carrots and cut them into the strips. Peel the potatoes and chop.

- Add the carrot strips and chopped potatoes in the slow cooker after 4 hours of cooking.

- Chop the fresh cilantro and add it in the slow cooker too.

- Stir the mix and close the slow cooker lid. Cook the stew for 3 hours more on LOW.

- Serve the prepared dish immediately or keep it in the fridge, not more than 3 days. Enjoy!

Nutrition: Calories 207, Fat 3.5, Fiber 8, Carbs 3.67, Protein 8

9. Carrot Soup with Cardamom

Preparation time: 18 minutes

Cooking time: 12 hours

Servings: 9

Ingredients:

- 1pound carrot
- 1teaspoon ground cardamom
- 1/4teaspoon nutmeg
- 1teaspoon salt
- 3tablespoons fresh parsley
- 1teaspoon honey
- 1teaspoon marjoram
- 5cups chicken stock
- 1/2cup yellow onion, chopped
- 1teaspoon butter

Directions:

1. Toss the butter in a pan and add chopped onion.
2. Chop the carrot and add it to the pan too.
3. Roast the vegetables for 5 minutes on the low heat. After this, place the roasted vegetables in the slow cooker. Add ground cardamom, nutmeg, salt, marjoram, and chicken stock.
4. Close the slow cooker lid and cook the soup for 12 hours on LOW.
5. Chop the fresh parsley.

6. When the time is over, blend the soup with a hand blender until you get a smooth texture. Then ladle the soup into the serving bowls.

7. Sprinkle the prepared soup with the chopped fresh parsley and honey. Enjoy the soup immediately!

Nutrition: Calories 80 Fat 2.7 Fiber 2, Carbs 1.19 Protein 4

10. Cod Chowder

Preparation time: 20 minutes

Cooking time: 3 hours

Servings: 6

Ingredients:

- yellow onion
- 10oz.. cod
- 3oz.. bacon, sliced
- 1teaspoon sage
- 5oz.. potatoes
- 1carrot, grated
- 5cups water
- 1tablespoon almond milk
- 1teaspoon ground coriander
- 1teaspoon salt

Directions:

1. Peel the onion and chop it.
2. Put the chopped onion and grated carrot in the slow cooker bowl. Add the sage, almond milk, ground coriander, and water. After this, chop the cod into the 6 pieces.
3. Add the fish in the slow cooker bowl too. Then chop the sliced bacon and peel the potatoes.
4. Cut the potatoes into the cubes.

5. Add the Ingredients: in the slow cooker bowl and close the slow cooker lid.

6. Cook the chowder for 3 hours on HIGH. Ladle the prepared cod chowder in the serving bowls.

7. Sprinkle the dish with the chopped parsley if desired. Enjoy!

Nutrition: Calories 108 Fat 4.5 Fiber 2, Carbs 3.02 Protein 10

11. Chicken Fajitas

Preparation Time: 10 minutes Cooking Time: 3 hours

Servings: 6

Ingredients:

- 11/2 lb.. chicken breast fillet
- 1/2cup salsa
- 2oz.. cream cheese
- 1teaspoon cumin
- 1teaspoon paprika
- Salt and pepper to taste
- 1onion, sliced
- 1clove garlic, minced
- 1red bell pepper, sliced
- 1green bell pepper, sliced
- 1teaspoon lime juice

Directions:

1. Combine all the ingredients except the lime wedges in your slow cooker. Cover the pot.
2. Cook on high for 3 hours.
3. Shred the chicken.
4. Drizzle with lime juice.
5. Serve with toppings like sour cream and cheese.

Nutrition: Calories 276 Fat 17 g Cholesterol 105 mg Sodium 827 mg Carbohydrate 3 g Protein 25 g Sugars 2 g

12. Tuscan Garlic Chicken

Preparation Time: 15 minutes

Cooking Time: 3 hours

Servings: 6

Ingredients:

- 1tablespoon Italian seasoning
- Salt and pepper to taste
- 1/2 cup sundried 1tablespoon olive oil
- 2cloves garlic, crushed and minced
- 1/2cup chicken broth
- 1cup heavy cream
- 3/4cup Parmesan cheese, grated
- 2chicken breasts tomatoes, chopped
- 2 cups spinach, chopped

Directions:

1. Pour the oil into your pan over medium heat.
2. Cook the garlic for 1 minute.
3. Stir in the broth and cream.
4. Simmer for 10 minutes.
5. Stir in the Parmesan cheese and remove from heat.
6. Put the chicken in your slow cooker.
7. Season with the salt, pepper and Italian seasoning.
8. Place the tomatoes on top of the chicken.
9. Pour the cream mixture on top of the chicken.
10. Cover the pot.

11. Cook on high for 3 hours.

12. Take the chicken out of the slow cooker and set aside

13. Add the spinach and stir until wilted.

14. Pour the sauce over the chicken and serve with the sun-dried tomatoes and spinach.

Nutrition: Calories 306 Fat 18.4g Cholesterol 115mg Sodium 287mg Carbohydrate 4.9g Protein 30.1g Sugars 2g

13.Balsamic Chicken

Preparation Time: 15 minutes

Cooking Time: 4 hours

Servings: 8

Ingredients

- 1tablespoon olive oil
- 2chicken breasts fillets
- 30oz.. canned diced tomatoes
- 1onion, sliced thinly
- 2cloves garlic
- 1/2cup balsamic vinegar
- 1teaspoon dried rosemary
- 1teaspoon dried basil
- 1teaspoon dried oregano
- 1/2teaspoon thyme
- Salt and pepper to taste

Directions:

1. Add the oil to your slow cooker.
2. Place the chicken breasts inside the pot.
3. Put the onions on top with the garlic cloves and herbs.
4. Pour the vinegar and tomatoes on top.
5. Cover the pot and cook on high for 4 hours.

Nutrition: Calories 238 Fat 12 g Cholesterol 73 mg Sodium 170 mg Carbohydrate 5 g Protein 25 g Sugars 4 g

14.Sesame Ginger Chicken

Preparation Time: 5 minutes

Cooking Time: 5 hours

Servings: 4

Ingredients:

- 11/2 lb.. chicken breast fillet
- 1/2cup tomato sauce
- 1/4cup low-sugar peach jam
- 1/4cup chicken broth
- 2tablespoons coconut amino
- 11/2 tablespoons sesame oil
- 1tablespoon honey
- 1teaspoon ground ginger
- 2cloves garlic, minced
- 1/4cup onion, minced
- 1/4teaspoon red pepper flakes, crushed
- 2tablespoons red bell pepper, chopped
- 11/2tablespoons green onion, chopped
- 2teaspoons sesame seeds

Directions:

1. Combine all the ingredients except green onion and sesame seeds in your slow cooker.
2. Mix well.
3. Cover the pot and cook on high for 4 hours.

4. Garnish with the green onion and sesame seeds.

Nutrition: Calories 220 Fat 13 g Sodium 246 mg Carbohydrate 7 g Protein 26 g Sugars 2 g

15.Ranch Chicken

Preparation Time: 5 minutes

Cooking Time: 4 hours and 5 minutes

Servings: 6

Ingredients:

- 2lb.. chicken breast fillet
- 2tablespoons butter
- 2oz.. cream cheese
- 3tablespoons ranch dressing mix

Directions:

1. Add the chicken to your slow cooker.
2. Place the butter and cream cheese on top of the chicken.
3. Sprinkle ranch dressing mix.
4. Seal the pot.
5. Cook on high for 4 hours.
6. Shred the chicken using forks and serve.

Nutrition: Calories 266 Fat 12.9 g Sodium 167 mg Potassium 450 mg Carbohydrate 4 g Fiber 0 g Protein 33 g Sugars 3 g

16.Chicken with Green Beans

Preparation Time: 5 minutes

Cooking Time: 4 hours

Servings: 4

Ingredients:

- 1onion, diced
- 2cloves garlic, crushed and minced
- 2tomatoes, diced
- 1/4cup dill, chopped
- 1lb.. green beans
- 1cup chicken broth
- 1tablespoon lemon juice
- 6chicken thighs
- Salt and pepper to taste
- 2tablespoons olive oil

Directions:

1. Put the onion, garlic, tomatoes, dill and green beans in your slow cooker.
2. Pour in the chicken broth and lemon juice.
3. Season with salt and pepper.
4. Mix well.
5. Add the chicken on top of the vegetables
6. Drizzle chicken with oil.
7. Cover the pot.

8. Cook on high for 4 hours.

Nutrition: Calories 373 Fat 26 g Sodium 315 mg Carbohydrate 1.4 g Fiber 4 g Protein 22 g Sugars 6 g

17.Greek Chicken

Preparation Time: 15 minutes

Cooking Time: 2 hours

Servings: 6

Ingredients:

- 2tablespoons olive oil
- 2cloves garlic
- 2lb.. chicken thigh fillets
- Salt and pepper to taste
- 1cup calamite olives
- 2oz.. marinated artichoke hearts, rinsed and drained
- 3oz.. roasted red peppers, drained and sliced
- 1onion, sliced
- 1/2cup chicken broth
- 1/4cup red wine vinegar
- 1tablespoon lemon juice
- 1teaspoon dried oregano
- 1teaspoon dried thyme
- 2tablespoons arrowroot starch

Directions:

1. Season the chicken with salt and pepper.
2. Put a pan over medium high heat.
3. Add the oil and garlic.
4. Cook for 1 minute, stirring frequently.

5. Add the chicken and cook for 2 minutes per side.

6. Transfer the chicken to the slow cooker.

7. Add the olives, artichoke hearts and peppers around the chicken.

8. Sprinkle onion on top.

9. In a bowl, mix the rest of the ingredients except the arrowroot starch.

10. Pour this into the slow cooker.

11. Cover the pot.

12. Cook on high for 2 hours.

13. Get 3 tablespoons of the cooking liquid.

14. Stir in the arrowroot starch to the liquid and put it back to the pot.

15. Simmer for 15 minutes before serving.

Nutrition: Calories 452 Fat 36 g Sodium 899 mg Carbohydrate 4 g Fiber 1 g Protein 26 g Sugars 3 g

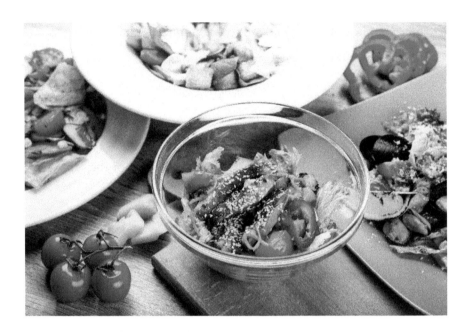

DINNER

18.Spinach Stuffed Portobello

Preparation Time: 15 minutes

Cooking Time: 3 hours

Servings: 8

Ingredients:

- 2 oz.. medium-sized Portobello mushrooms, stems removed
- 2 tablespoons olive oil
- 1/2 onion, chopped
- 2 cups fresh spinach, rinsed and chopped
- 3 garlic cloves, minced
- 1 cup chicken broth
- 3 tablespoons parmesan cheese, grated
- 1/3 teaspoon dried thyme
- Salt, pepper, to taste

Directions:

1. Heat oil in a medium pan over high heat.
2. Add onion, cook until translucent, stirring steadily. Add spinach and thyme, cook for 1-2 minutes until spinach is wilted.
3. Brush each mushroom with olive oil.

4. Put 1 tablespoon of onion and spinach stuffing into each mushroom.

5. Pour chicken broth into the slow cooker. Put stuffed mushrooms on the bottom.

6. Close the lid and cook on High for 3 hours.

7. Once cooked, sprinkle mushrooms with parmesan cheese and serve.

Nutrition: Calories 310g Fats 21g carbs 3g Protein 12g

19. Cod and Vegetables

Preparation Time: 15 minutes

Cooking Time: 1-3 hours

Servings: 4

Ingredients:

- 5-6 oz.. cod fillets
- 1 bell pepper, sliced or chopped
- 1 onion, sliced
- 1/2 fresh lemon, sliced
- 1 zucchini, sliced
- 3 garlic cloves, minced
- 1/4 cup low-sodium broth
- 1 teaspoon rosemary
- 1/4 teaspoon red pepper flakes
- Salt, pepper, to taste

Directions:

1. Season cod fillets with salt and pepper.
2. Pour broth into a slow cooker, add garlic, rosemary, bell pepper, onion, and zucchini into the slow cooker.
3. Put fish into your slow cooker, add lemon slices on top.
4. Close the lid and cook on Low for 2-3 hours or on High for 1 hour.

Nutrition: Calories 150 Fats 11.6g Carbs 2g Protein 26.9g

20. Balsamic Beef Pot Roast

Preparation Time: 15 minutes

Cooking Time: 4 hours

Servings: 10

Ingredients:

- 1boneless (3 lb..) chuck roast
- 1tbsp.Kosher salt
- 1tbsp Black ground pepper
- 1tbsp Garlic powder
- 1/4 cup balsamic vinegar
- 1/2 cup chopped onion
- 2cup. water
- 1/4 tsp. xanthan gum
- Fresh parsley for garnish

Directions:

1. Season the chuck roast with garlic powder, pepper, and salt over the entire surface.
2. Use a large skillet to sear the roast until browned.
3. Deglaze the bottom of the pot using balsamic vinegar. Cook one minute. Add to the slow cooker.
4. Mix in the onion and add the water. Once it starts to boil, secure the lid, and continue cooking on low for three to four hours.
5. Take the meat out of the slow cooker, and place it in a large bowl where you will break it up carefully into large chunks.

6. Remove all fat and anything else that may not be healthy, such as too much fat.

7. Whisk the xanthan gum into the broth and add it back to the slow cooker.

8. Serve and enjoy with a smile!

Nutrition: Calories: 393 Carbs: 3 g Protein: 30 g

21.Ribeye with Caramelized Onions and Mushrooms

Preparation Time: 15 minutes

Cooking Time: 15 minutes

Servings: 10

Ingredients:

- 2 (6-ounce) ribeye steaks
- 1tablespoon olive oil
- Salt
- Freshly ground black pepper
- 1/2tablespoons ghee or salted butter
- 1 yellow onion, sliced
- 1 cup sliced mushrooms

Directions:

1. Pat the steaks dry with paper towels, then rub them with the olive oil. Season generously with salt and pepper.
2. In a large skillet over medium heat, heat the butter. Add the onion and cook, stirring frequently, for 3 to 5 minutes, until it starts to soften. Add the mushrooms and cook until the mushrooms are tender and the onion is translucent, another 5 minutes or so. Transfer the mixture to a paper towel–lined plate.

3. In the skillet over medium-high heat, grill the steak for 4 to 5 minutes on each side, to your desired doneness. Plate the steaks and let rest for 5 minutes.

4. Serve the steak immediately with the mushrooms and onion spooned over the top.

Nutrition: Calories: 519; Protein: 52g; Carbs: 5g; Fiber: 1g;

22. **Beef Stroganoff**

Preparation Time: 5 minutes

Cooking Time: 20 minutes

Servings: 2

Ingredients:

- 1pound ground beef
- 1 tablespoon salted butter
- 1 yellow onion, diced
- 2cups mushrooms, sliced
- 1garlic cloves, minced
- 1 cup beef broth
- 1 cup sour cream
- 1/4 teaspoon xanthan gum
- Salt
- Freshly ground black pepper
- Chopped fresh parsley, for garnish (optional)
- Grated Parmesan cheese, for garnish (optional)

Directions:

1. In a large skillet over medium-high heat, cook the ground beef, stirring and breaking it up with a spatula, until cooked through, 7 to 10 minutes. Drain the fat and transfer the meat to a paper towel–lined plate.

2. In the same skillet still over medium-high heat, melt the butter. Add the onion, mushrooms, and garlic and cook, stirring

frequently, until the garlic is browned and the onion and mushrooms are tender, 5 to 7 minutes.

3. Add the broth, browned beef, sour cream, and xanthan gum to the skillet and cook, stirring, until the sauce is combined and thickened, 3 to 5 minutes.

4. Serve hot, garnished with the fresh parsley and grated Parmesan cheese (if using).

Directions: Calories: 369; Total Fat: 25g; Protein: 28g; Carbs: 5g;

23. Meatloaf

Preparation Time: 10 minutes

Cooking Time: 40 minutes

Servings: 4

Ingredients:

- 1pound ground beef
- 1 pound ground pork1
- large eggs
- 1 cup pork rinds, crushed
- 1/2 cup grated Parmesan cheese
- 1/4 cup heavy (whipping) cream
- 1 teaspoon prepared mustard
- Salt
- Freshly ground black pepper
- 1/4 cup sugar-free ketchup or tomato paste
- 1 tablespoon apple cider vinegar
- 1 teaspoon sugar substitute (such as Swerve)

Directions:

1. Preheat the oven to 400F. Line a sheet pan with aluminum foil.

2. In large bowl, combine the beef, pork, eggs, pork rinds, cheese, cream, and mustard, and season with salt and pepper. Stir to mix well.

3. Form the mixture into a loaf shape on the prepared sheet pan.

4. In a small bowl, stir together the ketchup, vinegar, and sweetener. Brush the mixture on top of the formed loaf.

5. Bake for 35 to 40 minutes, or until nicely browned with an internal temperature of 160°F.

6. Remove from the oven and let rest for 5 to 10 minutes before slicing and serving.

Nutrition: Calories: 465; Fat: 32g; Protein: 41g; Carbs: 1g;

24. Flank Steak and Broccoli

Preparation Time: 10 minutes

Cooking Time: 30 minutes

Servings: 4

Ingredients:

- 1pound flank steak
- 6 tablespoons olive oil, divided
- 1 teaspoon garlic powder
- 1 teaspoon onion powder
- Salt
- Freshly ground black pepper
- 4 cups broccoli florets

Directions:

1. In a large, resealable plastic bag, combine the steak and 3 tablespoons of olive oil with the garlic powder and onion powder. Season with salt and pepper. Refrigerate for at least 30 minutes, or up to 24 hours.

2. Set the oven broiler to high. Line a sheet pan with aluminum foil.

3. Place the steak and broccoli on the prepared sheet pan. Drizzle the remaining 3 tablespoons of olive oil over the broccoli, and season with salt and pepper. Toss until coated.

4. Cook under the broiler for 3 to 5 minutes, then flip the steak and continue to cook for 3 to 5 minutes more, or until the steak reaches your preferred doneness.

5. Let the steak rest for 10 minutes, then slice it thinly across the grain and serve with the roasted broccoli on the side.

Nutrition: Calories: 380; Fat: 30g; Protein: 26g; Carbs: 5g;

25. Barbecue Spare Ribs

Preparation Time: 15 minutes

Cooking Time: 5 hrs.

Servings: 5

Ingredients:

- 2 pounds spare ribs
- 1/2tablespoon salt
- 1 tablespoon garlic powder
- 1 tablespoon onion powder
- 1 tablespoon paprika
- 1 teaspoon ground cumin
- 1 teaspoon freshly ground black pepper

Directions:

1. Pat the ribs dry with paper towels, and slice them into sections to fit in the slow cooker.

2. In a small bowl, stir together the salt, garlic powder, onion powder, paprika, cumin, and pepper. Rub the seasoning mixture all over the ribs.

3. Place the ribs in the slow cooker and cook on low for 8 to 10 hours or on high for 4 to 5 hours, until the meat is very tender and falling off the bones.

4. Serve hot.

Nutrition: Calories: 263g; Fat: 19g; Protein: 21g; Carbs: 1g; Fiber: 0g

26.   Slow Cooker Pork Chili Colorado

Preparation Time: 10 minutes

Cooking Time: 8 hrs.

Servings: 8

Ingredients:

- 2 pounds boneless pork shoulder, cut into 1-inch cubes
- 1onion, chopped
- 1/2tablespoons chili powder
- 1 tablespoon chipotle chili powder
- 1 teaspoon sea salt
- Juice of 1 lime
- 1 avocado, cubed
- 1/2 cup grated Monterey Jack cheese
- 1/2 cup sour cream
- 1/4 cup chopped, fresh cilantro
- 6 green onions, sliced

Directions:

1. In a slow cooker, combine the pork shoulder, onion, chili powder, chipotle, and salt. Cover and cook on low for eight to ten hours, until the pork is soft.
2. Stir in the lime juice.
3. Serve garnished with the avocado, cheese, sour cream, cilantro, and onion.

Nutrition: Calories: 451;Fat: 33gProtein: 32g; Carbs: 5g; Fiber: 3g;

27. Thyme Sea Bass

Preparation Time: 15 minutes

Cooking Time: 15 minutes

Servings: 10

Ingredients:

- 11 oz. sea bass, trimmed
- 2 tablespoons coconut cream
- 3 oz. spring onions, chopped
- 1 teaspoon fennel seeds
- 1/2 teaspoon dried thyme
- 1 teaspoon olive oil
- 1/3 cup water
- 1 teaspoon apple cider vinegar
- 1/2 teaspoon salt

Directions:

1. In the slow cooker, mix the sea bass with the cream and the other ingredients.
2. Close the lid and cook sea bass for 4 hours on Low.

Nutrition: Calories 304, Fat 11.4, Fiber 0.9, Carbs 2.6,Protein 0.7

28. Butter-dipped Lobsters

Preparation Time: 15 minutes

Cooking Time: 1 hour

Servings: 3

Ingredients:

- 4 lb. lobster tails, cut in half

- 4 tablespoons of unsalted butter, melted

- Salt to taste

- Black pepper to taste

Directions:

1. Start by throwing all the Ingredients: into your Slow cooker.

2. Cover its lid and cook for 1 hour on Low setting.

3. Once done, remove its lid and give it a stir.

4. Serve warm.

Nutrition: Calories 324 Fat 20.7 g Carbs 3.6 g Sugar 1.4 g Fiber 0.5 g Protein 15.3 g

29. Fish And Salsa Bowl

Preparation Time: 15 minutes

Cooking Time: 2 hrs.

Servings: 6

Ingredients:

- 1-pound white fish fillets, boneless and cubed
- 1 cup keto salsa
- 1/2 teaspoon Italian seasoning
- 1/2 cup red cabbage, shredded
- 1/2 teaspoon paprika
- 2 tablespoons olive oil
- 1 tablespoon chives, chopped

Directions:

1. In the slow cooker, mix the fish with the salsa and the other ingredients.
2. Close the lid and cook on High for 2 hours.
3. Divide into bowls and serve.

Nutrition: Calories 238, Fat 16.3, Fiber 1.9, Carbs 5 Protein 11.8

30. Shrimp Chowder

Preparation time: 15 minutes

Cooking time: 1 Hour

Servings: 4

Ingredients

- 1-pound shrimps
- ½ cup fennel bulb, chopped
- 1 bay leaf
- ½ teaspoon peppercorn
- 1 cup of coconut milk
- cups of water
- 1 teaspoon ground coriander

Directions:

1 Put all Ingredients: in the Slow Cooker.

2 Close the lid and cook the chowder on High for 1 hour.

Nutrition: 277 calories, 27.4g protein, 6.1g carbohydrates, 16.3g fat, 1.8g fiber, 239mg cholesterol, 297mg sodium, 401mg potassium.

31. Ground Pork Soup

Preparation time: 15 minutes

Cooking time: 5.5 Hour

Servings: 4

Ingredients

- 1 cup ground pork
- ½ cup red kidney beans, canned
- 1 cup tomatoes, canned
- cups of water
- 1 tablespoon dried cilantro
- 1 teaspoon salt

Directions:

1 Put ground pork in the Slow Cooker.

2 Add tomatoes, water, dried cilantro, and salt. Close the lid and cook the Ingredients: on High for 5 hours.

3 Then add canned red kidney beans and cook the soup on high for 30 minutes more.

Nutrition: 318 calories, 25.7g protein, 10.9g carbohydrates, 16.6g fat, 4.1g fiber, 74mg cholesterol, 651mg sodium, 706mg potassium.

MEAT RECIPES

32.   Split Peas with Ham

Preparation time: 10 minutes

Cooking time: 8 hours

Servings: 8

Ingredients:

- 1 medium onion, chopped
- 4 medium carrots, diced
- 8 medium ham hocks, about 4 ounces each
- 2½ quarts boiling water
- 1-pound dry yellow split peas
- Salt and Pepper

Directions:

1   Bring water to a boil in a saucepan.

2   Place ingredients into a slow cooker.

3   Add boiling water and stir together.

4   Cover and cook on HIGH for 4 hours or on LOW for 7-8 hours until vegetables are tender.

5   Remove the ham hocks from the slow cooker when cooked. Debone the meat. Stir cut-up chunks of meat back into the slow cooker before serving.

Nutrition: calories 271, fat 18, carbs 23, protein 28

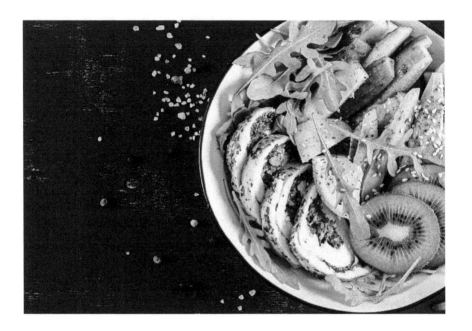

POULTRY

33. Rotisserie Chicken

Preparation Time: 10 minutes

Cooking Time: 8 hours 5 minutes

Servings: 10

Ingredients:

- 1 organic whole chicken
- 1 tablespoon of olive oil
- 1 teaspoon of thyme
- 1 teaspoon of rosemary
- 1 teaspoon of garlic, granulated
- salt and pepper

Directions:

1. Start by seasoning the chicken with all the herbs and spices.
2. Broil this seasoned chicken for 5 minutes in the oven until golden brown.
3. Place this chicken in the Slow cooker.
4. Cover it and cook for 8 hours on Low Settings.
5. Serve warm.

Nutrition: Calories 301 Total Fat 12.2 g Saturated Fat 2.4 g Cholesterol 110 mg Total Carbs 2.5 g Fiber 0.9 g Sugar 1.4 g Sodium 276 mg Potassium 231 mg Protein 28.8 g

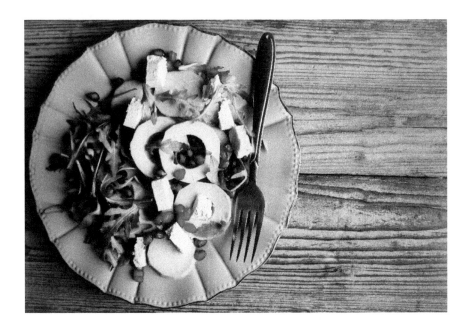

SIDE DISH RECIPES

34. Green Beans and Mushrooms

Preparation time: 15 minutes

Cooking time: 3 Hours

Servings: 4

Ingredients

- 1 pound fresh green beans, trimmed
- 1 small yellow onion, chopped
- 6 ounces bacon, chopped
- 1 garlic clove, minced
- 1 cup chicken stock
- 8 ounces mushrooms, sliced
- Salt and black pepper to the taste
- A splash of balsamic vinegar

Directions:

1. In your Slow cooker, mix beans with onion, bacon, garlic, stock, mushrooms, salt, pepper and vinegar, stir, cover and cook on Low for 3 hours.
2. Divide between plates and serve as a side dish.

Nutrition: calories 162, fat 4, fiber 5, carbs 8, protein 4

35.   Beans and Red Peppers

Preparation time: 15 minutes

Cooking time: 2 Hrs.

Servings: 2

Ingredients

- 2 cups green beans, halved
- 1 red bell pepper, cut into strips
- Salt and black pepper to the taste
- 1 tbsp. olive oil
- 1 and ½ tbsp. honey mustard

Directions:

1. Add green beans; honey mustard, red bell pepper, oil, salt, and black to Slow cooker.
2. Put on the cooker's lid on and set the cooking time to hours on High settings.
3. Serve warm.

Nutrition: Per Serving: Calories: 50, Total Fat: 0g, Fiber: 4g, Total Carbs: 8g, Protein: 2g

VEGETABLES

36. Zucchini and Yellow Squash

Preparation time: 15 minutes

Cooking time: 6 hours

Servings: 2

Ingredients

- 2/3 cup zucchini, sliced
- 2/3 cups yellow squash, sliced
- 1/3 tsp Italian seasoning
- 1/8 cup butter

Directions:

1. Place zucchini and squash on the bottom of the slow cooker.
2. Sprinkle with the Italian seasoning with salt, pepper, and garlic powder to taste. Top with butter.
3. Cover and cook within 6 hours on low.

Nutrition: Calories: 122 Fat: 9.9 g Carbs: 3.7 g Protein: 4.2 g

37.   Gluten-Free Zucchini Bread

Preparation time: 15 minutes

Cooking time: 3 hours

Servings: 2

Ingredients

- 1/2 cup coconut flour
- 1/2 tsp baking powder and baking soda
- 1egg, whisked
- 1/4 cup butter
- 1cup zucchini, shredded

Directions:

1. Combine all dry Ingredients: and add a pinch of salt and sweetener of choice. Combine the dry Ingredients: with the eggs and mix thoroughly.
2. Fold in zucchini and spread inside the slow cooker. Cover and cook within 3 hours on high.

Nutrition: Calories: 174 Fat: 13 g Carbs: 2.9 g Protein: 4 g

38. Eggplant Parmesan

Preparation time: 40 minutes

Cooking time: 4 hours

Servings: 2

Ingredients

- 1large eggplant, 1/2-inch slices
- 1egg, whisked
- 1tsp Italian seasoning
- 1cup marinara
- 1/4 cup Parmesan cheese, grated

Directions:

1. Put salt on each side of the eggplant, then let stand for 30 minutes.

2. Spread some of the marinara on the bottom of the slow cooker and season with salt and pepper, garlic powder, and Italian seasoning.

3. Spread the eggplants on a single the slow cooker and pour over some of the marinara sauce. Repeat up to 3 layers. Top with Parmesan. Cover and cook for 4 hours.

Nutrition: Calories: 159 Fat: 12 g Carbs: 8 g Protein: 14 g

39. Zucchini Lasagna

Preparation time: 15 minutes

Cooking time: 4 hours

Servings: 2

Ingredients

- 1large egg, whisked
- 1/8 cup Parmesan cheese, grated
- 1cup spinach, chopped
- 2cups tomato sauce
- 2zucchinis, 1/8-inch thick, pre-grilled

Directions:

1. Mix egg with spinach and parmesan. Spread some of the tomato sauce inside the slow cooker and season with salt and pepper.
2. Spread the zucchini on a single the slow cooker and pour over some of the tomato sauce. Repeat until 3 layers.
3. Top with Parmesan.
4. Cover and cook for 4 hours.

Nutrition: Calories: 251 Fat: 13.9 g Carbs: 4.8 g Protein: 20.8 g

40. Cauliflower Bolognese on Zucchini Noodles

Preparation time: 15 minutes

Cooking time: 4 hours

Servings: 2

Ingredients

- 1cauliflower head, floret cuts
- 1tsp dried basil flakes
- 28oz. diced tomatoes
- 1/2 cup vegetable broth
- 5zucchinis, spiral cut

Directions:

1 Place Ingredients: in the slow cooker except for the zucchini. Season with 2 garlic cloves, 3.4 diced onions, salt, pepper to taste, and desired spices. Cover and cook for 4 hours.

2 Smash florets of the cauliflower with a fork to form "Bolognese."

3 Transfer the dish on top of the zucchini noodles.

Nutrition: Calories: 164 Fat: 5 g Carbs: 6 g Protein: 12 g

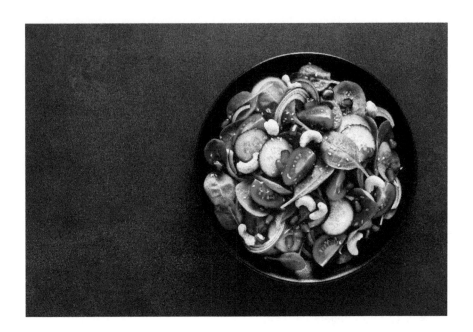

FISH & SEAFOOD

41.Shrimp Bake

Preparation Time: 10 minutes

Cooking time: 2 hours

Servings: 2

Ingredients:

- `1-pound shrimp, peeled and deveined
- `2 tablespoons lime juice
- `1 teaspoon salt
- `1 teaspoon apple cider vinegar
- `1 tablespoon butter
- `¾ cup heavy cream
- `2 oz provolone cheese, shredded

Directions:

1   In the slow cooker, mix the shrimp with the lime juice and the other ingredients except the cheese.

2   Toss, sprinkle the cheese on top, and cook on High for 2 hours.

Nutrition: calories 290, fat 5, carbs 3, protein 18

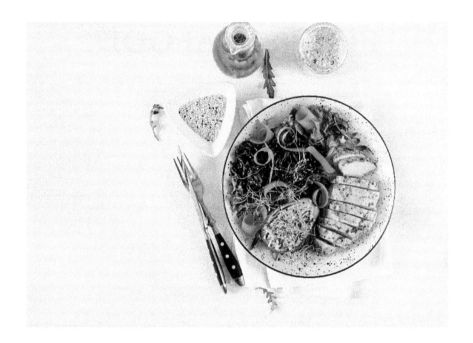

APPETIZERS & SNACKS

42. Savory Pine Nuts Cabbage

Preparation Time: 10 minutes

Cooking Time: 2 hours

Servings: 2

Ingredients:

- 1savoy cabbage, shredded
- 2tablespoons of avocado oil
- 1tablespoon of balsamic vinegar
- 1/4cup of pine nuts, toasted
- 1/2cup of vegetable broth
- Salt and black pepper- to taste

Directions:

1. Start by throwing all the Ingredients: into the Slow cooker.
2. Cover its lid and cook for 2 hours on Low setting.
3. Once done, remove its lid of the slow cooker carefully.
4. Mix well and garnish as desired.
5. Serve warm.

Nutrition: Calories 145 Fat 13.1 g Sodium 35 mg Carbs 4 g Sugar 1.2 g Fiber 1.5 g Protein 3.5 g

43.   Plantains with Tapioca Pearls

Preparation Time: 15 Minutes Cooking Time: 3 Hours

Servings: 6

Ingredients:

- 5ripe plantains, sliced into thick disks
- 1can thick coconut cream
- 1tsp.. coconut oil
- 1/4cup tiny tapioca pearls, dried
- 1cup white sugar
- 2cups water
- Pinch of salt

Directions:

1. Grease the Instant Pot Pressure Cooker with coconut oil.

2. Place ripe plantains. Top this with tapioca pearls, coconut oil, white sugar, and salt. Pour just the right amount of water into the Instant Pot.

3. Lock the lid in place. Press the high pressure and cook for 5 minutes.

4. When the beep sounds, Choose the Quick Pressure Release. This will depressurize for 7 minutes. Remove the lid.

5. Tip in in coconut cream. Allow residual heat cook the last ingredient.

6. To serve, ladle just the right amount of plantains into dessert bowls.

Nutrition: Calories 345 Fat 8 Fiber 4.5 Carbs 3.5 Protein 20

44.   Mango Cashew Cake

Preparation Time: 15 Minutes

Cooking Time: 1 hour

Servings: 8

Ingredients:

- 1/4tsp.. coconut oil, for greasing
- 1tsp.. baking powder
- 1/2tsp.. baking soda
- 1/4cup coconut butter
- 1Tbsp.. flour
- 1/2cup all-purpose flour
- 1/4cup mango jam
- 1/2cup cashew milk
- 1/4cup ground cashew nuts
- 1tsp.. vanilla essence
- 1/2cup powdered sugar
- 21/2 cups water

Directions:

1. Lightly grease the Instant Pot Pressure Cooker with coconut oil. Dust with flour. Set aside.

2. Meanwhile, combine all-purpose flour, coconut butter, baking powder, cashew milk, baking soda, vanilla essence, mango jam, and cashew nuts in a large mixing bowl. Stir until all ingredients come together. Pour batter on a Bundt pan.

3. Place trivet on pressure cooker. Pour 2 1/2 cups of water.

4. Lock the lid in place. Press the high pressure and cook for 35 minutes.

5. When the beep sounds, Choose Natural Pressure Release. Depressurizing would take 20 minutes. Remove the lid.

6. Take out Bundt cake. Transfer to a cake rack. Let cool for 10 minutes at room temperature.

7. Turn cake over on a serving dish. Sprinkle powdered sugar. Slice and serve.

Nutrition: Calories 213 Fat 21 Fiber 5 Carbs 1.9 Protein 21

45. Sweet Orange and Lemon Barley Risotto

Preparation Time: 5 Minutes

Cooking Time: 45 minutes

Servings: 4

Ingredients:

- 11/2cups barley pearls
- 1/4cup raisins
- 1cup sweet orange, chopped, reserve juice
- 4cups water
- 4strips lemon peels
- 1/4cup white sugar, add more if needed

Directions:

1. Combine barley pearls, lemon peels, raisins, water, and white sugar into the Instant Pot Pressure Cooker.
2. Lock the lid in place. Press the high pressure and cook for 10 minutes.
3. When the beep sounds, Choose the Quick Pressure Release. This will depressurize for 7 minutes. Remove the lid. Discard lemon peels.
4. Add in sweet orange and juices. Pour coconut cream. Allow residual heat cook the coconut cream. Adjust seasoning according to your preferred taste.
5. To serve, ladle equal amounts into dessert bowls. Cool slightly before serving.

Nutrition: Calories 124 Fat 11 Fiber 15 Carbs 3.9 Protein 28

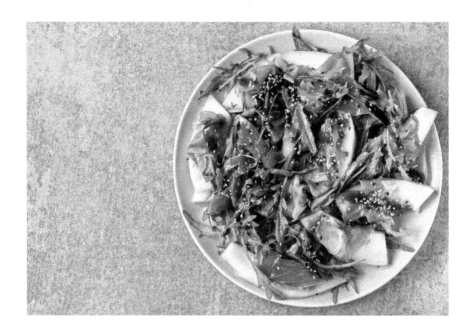

DESSERT

46.   Luscious Walnut Chocolate Brownies

Preparation Time: 30 minutes

Cooking Time 55 minutes

Servings: 6-8

Ingredients:

- `180 g pitted dates

- `30 ml water

- `6 tbsp.. salted butter

- `210 g chopped dark chocolate

- `2 eggs (l)

- `2 tbsp.. cocoa powder

- `2 tbsp.. whole meal spelled flour

- `130 g California walnuts (roughly chopped)

- `2 tbsp.. powdered sugar

Directions:

1. Preheat the oven to 180 degrees. Grease a rectangular baking pan (23 cm) and line it with baking paper.

2. Put dates and water in a blender and puree to a paste. Put aside.

3. Melt the butter and chocolate in a large pan while stirring. Take the pan off the heat, let the chocolate cool down a bit

and then stir in the date paste. Then gradually stir in the eggs carefully. Sift the cocoa and flour into a bowl, then add to the pan and mix with a wooden spoon to form a smooth batter.

4. Add walnuts to the dough, mix in and then pour the dough into the prepared baking pan. Then bake for 20 to 25 minutes until the brownie batter is firm in the middle. Then let cool down completely. Then decorate with a little icing sugar and a stencil.

Nutrition: Calories 214 Fat 3 Fiber 3 Carbs 2.5 Protein 8

47. Gluten-free Chocolate Cake

Preparation Time: 40 minutes

Cooking Time 1 hour and 30 minutes

Servings: 6-8

Ingredients:

- `200 g dark chocolate coverture (gluten-free)
- `200 g butter
- `150 g whole cane sugar
- `5 eggs
- `100 g ground almond
- `2 tsp.. baking powder
- `250 g potato starch
- `250 g cornmeal
- `40 g cocoa powder

Directions:

1. Roughly chop the coverture with a knife. Melt over a hot water bath and allow cooling.

2. Mix butter with sugar in a bowl until frothy. Gradually stir in eggs until a creamy mixture is formed. Stir liquid chocolate, almonds, baking powder, starch, cornflour, and cocoa into the foam mixture.

3. Line the baking sheet with parchment paper. Spread the dough on the baking sheet and bake in the preheated oven at 180C for about 25–30 minutes. Make a chopstick test.

Nutrition: Calories 312 Fat 5 Fiber 8 Carbs 4.6 Protein 12

48.   Brownies with Nuts

Preparation Time: 30 minutes

Cooking Time 45 minutes

Servings: 6-8

Ingredients:

- `250 g soft butter
- `150 g sugar
- `4 eggs
- `200 g dark chocolate
- `250 g ground hazelnuts
- `250 g flour
- `1/2 tsp.. baking powder
- `1/2 tsp.. cinnamon
- `1 tbsp.. cocoa powder
- `For covering
- `250 g butter
- `250 g sugar
- `800 g condensed milk
- `120 g honey
- `600 g mixed nuts

Directions:

1. Preheat the oven to 200 C top and bottom heat.
2. Mix the butter with the sugar and the eggs until creamy. Grate the chocolate and stir into the butter-egg mixture with the

ground nuts, flour, baking powder, cinnamon, and cocoa. Spread the dough about 2 cm thick on a greased baking sheet and bake in the preheated oven for 20-25 minutes.

3. For the topping, heat the butter, add the sugar and condensed milk, mix in the honey, bring to a boil and simmer for 5-10 minutes, stirring, until everything is caramelized. Fold in the coarsely chopped, mixed nuts, pour over the finished brownie batter, spread on, and let cool. Serve cut into small rectangles.

Nutrition: Calories 234 Fat 8 Fiber 6 Carbs 1.3 Protein 15

49. Halloween Brownies

Preparation Time: 30 minutes

Cooking Time 1 hour 45 minutes

Servings: 8

Ingredients:

- `600 g Hokkaido pumpkin
- `75 g whole cane sugar
- `1 tsp.. cinnamon powder
- `1/2 tsp.. ginger powder
- `1 pinch ground mace
- `200 g dark chocolate (at least 70% cocoa content)
- `90 g agave syrup
- `1/2 tsp.. vanilla powder
- `175 g room temperature butter
- `1 pinch salt
- `5 eggs
- `100 g spelled flour type 1050
- `1 tbsp.. baking powder
- `50 g cocoa powder
- `200 g cream cheese

Directions:

1. Cut the calf, cut half, center, and wedge the pulp. In a bakery boiler with a bakery, cover the pumpkin and baker for about 40 minutes in a preheated oven at 200 C

2. Take the kitchen, fine puree, cinnamon, ginger, and mace, all with whole cane sugar, and allow to cool..

3. Cut the chocolate roughly into it and melt it over a bath of hot water.

4. Mix agave powder, butter, and salt in the mixture with agave syrup to creamy. Remove in 3 eggs one by one. Chocolate subject. Mix meal, baking powder, and cocoa powder and then add chocolate and agave syrup carefully. In the mould, add the mixture and smooth.

5. With cream cheese, mix the pumpkin puree and the rest of the eggs. Put into the mould the mixture of the pumpkin and cream cheese and sprinkle it onto the chocolate with a wood spoon.

6. Bake for 30–35 minutes in the oven at 200 degrees C (fan oven 180 degrees C, gas level 3). Take it out, let it cool, cut it in pieces.

Nutrition: Calories 342 Fat 6 Fiber 3 Carbs 2.9 Protein 9

50. Raw Brownies with Cashew Nuts

Preparation Time: 30 minutes

Cooking Time 1 hour 45 minutes

Servings: 8

Ingredients:

- `450 g dried dates
- `150 g cashew nuts
- `300 g ground almond kernels
- `110 g cocoa powder (heavily de-oiled)
- `45 g almond flour (3 tbsp..)
- `1 pinch salt
- `1/2 vanilla pod

Directions:

1. Just cover the dates with water and leave to soak overnight. On the next day, pour off the date water, put it on top, and set aside. Puree the softened dates with a hand blender to a creamy paste and add some date water if necessary, so that the mixture becomes creamy.

2. Chop the cashew nuts. Halve the vanilla pod lengthways, scrape out the pulp. Mix the almonds, cocoa, almond flour, 100 g cashew nuts, 1 pinch of salt, and vanilla pulp in a bowl, and knead with the date paste.

3. Pour the dough into a baking dish or baking tin (30 x 20 cm) lined with baking paper and press firmly.

4. Let the dough set in the refrigerator for at least 4 hours. Then cut into 15 pieces and decorate with the remaining cashew nuts.

Nutrition: Calories 342 Fat 8 Fiber 5 Carbs 1.9 Protein 9

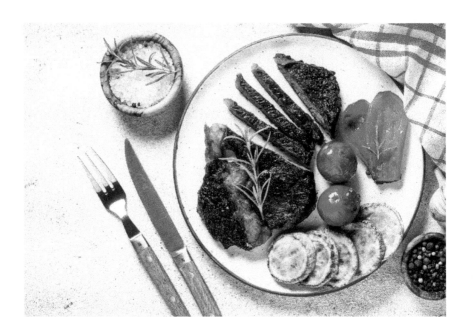

30 DAY MEAL PLAN

DAY	BREAKFAST	LUNCH	DINNER	DESSERTS
1	Egg Sausage Breakfast Casserole	Garlic Duck Breast	Pork Chops	Chocolate Mousse
2	Vegetable Omelet	Thyme Lamb Chops	Spicy Pork & Spinach Stew	Chocolate Chia Pudding With Almonds
3	Cheese Bacon Quiche	Autumn Pork Stew	Stuffed Taco Peppers	Coconut Macadamia Chia Pudding
4	Egg Breakfast Casserole	Handmade Sausage Stew	Chinese Pulled Pork	Keto Chocolate Mug
5	Cauliflower Breakfast Casserole	Marinated Beef Tenderloin	Bacon Wrapped Pork Loin	Vanilla Chia Pudding
6	Veggie Frittata	Chicken Liver Sauté	Lamb Barbacoa	Choco Lava Cake
7	Feta Spinach Quiche	Chicken In Bacon	Balsamic Pork Tenderloin	Coconut Cup Cakes
8	Cauliflower Mashed	Whole Chicken	Spicy Pork	Easy Chocolate Cheesecake
9	Kalua Pork With Cabbage	Duck Rolls	Zesty Garlic Pulled Pork	Chocolate Chip Brownie
10	Creamy Pork	Keto Adobo	Ranch	Coconut

	Chops	Chicken	Pork Chops	Cookies
11	Beef Taco Filling	Cayenne Pepper Drumsticks	Pork Chile Verde	Choco Pie
12	Flavorful Steak Fajitas	Keto Bbq Chicken Wings	Ham Soup	Keto Blueberry Muffins
13	Garlic Herb Pork	Sweet Corn Pilaf	Beef And Broccoli	Keto Oven-Baked Brie Cheese
14	Garlic Thyme Lamb Chops	Mediterranean Vegetable Mix	Korean Barbecue Beef	Keto Vanilla Pound Cake
15	Pork Tenderloin	Spaghetti Cottage Cheese Casserole	Garlic Chicken	Almond Roll With Pumpkin Cream Cheese Filling
16	Smoky Pork With Cabbage	Meatballs With Coconut Gravy	Lamb Shanks	No Bake Low Carb Lemon Strawberry Cheesecake
17	Italian Frittata	Fresh Dal	Jamaican Jerk Pork Roast	Pecan Cheesecake
18	Easy Mexican Chicken	Pulled Pork Salad	Salmon	Blueberry And Zucchini Muffins
19	Cherry Tomatoes Thyme	Garlic Pork Belly	Coconut Chicken	Coffee Mousse

	Asparagus Frittata			
20	Healthy Veggie Omelet	Sesame Seed Shrimp	Mahi Mahi Taco Wraps	Chocolate Cake
21	Scrambled Eggs With Smoked Salmon	Chicken Liver Pate	Shrimp Tacos	Sweet Potato Brownies
22	Persian Omelet Slow cooker	Cod Fillet In Coconut Flakes	Fish Curry	Raspberry Brownies
23	Keto Slow cooker Tasty Onions	Prawn Stew	Salmon With Creamy Lemon Sauce	Brownie Cheesecake
24	Crustless Slow cooker Spinach Quiche	Pork-Jalapeno Bowl	Salmon With Lemon-Caper Sauce	Zucchini-Brownies
25	Eggplant Pate With Breadcrumbs	Chicken Marsala	Spicy Barbecue Shrimp	Bean Brownies
26	Red Beans With The Sweet Peas	Chickpeas Soup	Lemon Dill Halibut	Luscious Walnut Chocolate Brownies
27	Nutritious Burrito Bowl	Hot And Delicious Soup	Coconut Cilantro Curry Shrimp	Gluten-Free Chocolate Cake
28	Quinoa Curry	Delicious	Shrimp In	Brownies

		Eggplant Salad	Marinara Sauce	With Nuts
29	Ham Pitta Pockets	Tasty Black Beans Soup	Garlic Shrimp	Halloween Brownies
30	Breakfast Meatloaf	Rich Sweet Potato Soup	Lemon Pepper Tilapia	Raw Brownies With Cashew Nuts

CONVERSION TABLES

Volume Equivalents (Liquid)

US STANDARD	US STANDARD (OUNCES)	METRIC (APPROXIMATE)
2 tablespoons	1 fl. oz...	30 mL
1/4 cup	2 fl. oz...	60 mL
1/2 cup	4 fl. oz...	120 mL
1 cup	8 fl. oz...	240 mL
11/2 cups	12 fl. oz...	355 mL
2 cups or 1 pint	16 fl. oz...	475 mL
4 cups or 1 quart	32 fl. oz...	1 L
1 gallon	128 fl. oz...	4 L

Volume Equivalents (Dry)

US STANDARD	METRIC (APPROXIMATE)
1/4 teaspoon	1 mL
1/2 teaspoon	2 mL
1 teaspoon	5 mL
1 tablespoon	15 mL
1/4 cup	59 mL
cup	79 mL
1/2 cup	118 mL
1 cup	177 mL

Oven Temperatures

FAHRENHEIT (F)	CELSIUS (C) (APPROXIMATE)
250°F	120 °C
300°F	150°C
325°F	165°C
350°F	180°C
375°F	190°C
400°F	200°C
425°F	220°C
450°F	230°C

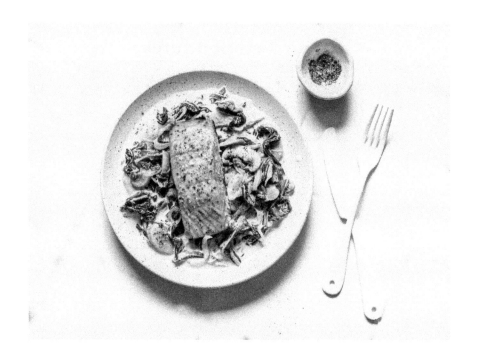

CONCLUSION

N
ow you can cook healthier meals for yourself, your family, and your friends that will get your metabolism running at the peak of perfection and will help you feel healthy, lose weight, and maintain a healthy balanced diet. A new diet isn't so bad when you have so many options from which to choose. You may miss your carbs, but with all these tasty recipes at your fingertips, you'll find them easily replaced with new favorites.

You will marvel at how much energy you have after sweating though the first week or so of almost no carbs. It can be a challenge, but you can do it! Pretty soon you won't miss those things that bogged down your metabolism as well as your thinking and made you tired and cranky. You will feel like you can rule the world and do anything, once your body is purged of heavy carbs and you start eating things that rejuvenate your body. It is worth the few detox symptoms when you actually start enjoying the food you are eating.

A Keto diet isn't one that you can keep going on and off. It will take your body some time to get adjusted and for ketosis to set in. This process could take anywhere between two to seven days. It is dependent on the level of activity, your body type and the food that you are eating.

There are various mobile applications that you can make use of for tracking your carbohydrate intake. There are paid and free applications as well. These apps will help you in keeping a track of your total carbohydrate and fiber intake. However, you won't be able to track your net carb intake. MyFitnessPal is one of the popular apps. You just need to open the app store on your smartphone, and you can select an app from the various apps that are available.

The amount of weight that you will lose will depend on you. If you add exercise to your daily routine, then the weight loss will be greater. If you cut down on foods that stall weight loss, then this will speed up the process. For instance, completely cutting out things like artificial sweeteners, dairy and wheat products and other related products will definitely help in speeding up your weight loss. During the first two weeks of the Keto diet, you will end up losing all the excess water weight. Ketosis has a diuretic effect on the body, and you might end up losing a couple of pounds within the first few days of this diet. After this, your body will adapt itself to burning fats for generating energy, instead of carbs.

You now have everything you need to break free from a dependence on highly processed foods, with all their dangerous additives that your body interprets as toxins. Today, when you want a sandwich for lunch, you'll roll the meat in Swiss cheese or a lettuce leaf and won't miss the bread at all, unless that is, you've made up the Keto bread recipe you discovered in this book! You can still enjoy your favorite pasta dishes, even taco salad, but without the grogginess in the afternoon that comes with all those unnecessary carbs.

So, energize your life and sustain a healthy body by applying what you've discovered. You don't have to change everything at once. Just start by adopting a new recipe each week that sounds interesting to you. Gradually, swap out less-than-healthy options for ingredients and recipes from this book that will promote your well-being.

Each time you make a healthy substitution or try a new ketogenic recipe, you can feel proud of yourself; you are actually taking good care of your mind and body. Even before you start to experience the benefits of a ketogenic lifestyle, you can feel good because you are choosing the best course for your life.

Thanks for reading.

Lightning Source UK Ltd.
Milton Keynes UK
UKHW022025010321
379617UK00008B/154